Yoga: Breathe, Move, Meditate

Yoga: Breathe, Move, Meditate

"Don't Let the Bed Get You"

Mary Ann Gullo (M.A.G.)

BALBOA.
PRESS

A DIVISION OF HAY HOUSE

Balboa Press books may be ordered through booksellers or by contacting:

Balboa Press
A Division of Hay House
1663 Liberty Drive
Bloomington, IN 47403
www.balboapress.com
1-(877) 407-4847

Because of the dynamic nature of the Internet, any web addresses or
links contained in this book may have changed since publication and
may no longer be valid. The views expressed in this work are solely those
of the author and do not necessarily reflect the views of the publisher,
and the publisher hereby disclaims any responsibility for them.

The author of this book does not dispense medical advice or prescribe the use
of any technique as a form of treatment for physical, emotional, or medical
problems without the advice of a physician, either directly or indirectly. The
intent of the author is only to offer information of a general nature to help you
in your quest for emotional and spiritual well-being. In the event you use any
of the information in this book for yourself, which is your constitutional right,
the author and the publisher assume no responsibility for your actions.

Any people depicted in stock imagery provided by Thinkstock are models,
and such images are being used for illustrative purposes only.
Certain stock imagery © Thinkstock.

Printed in the United States of America.

ISBN: 978-1-4525-7512-4 (sc)
ISBN: 978-1-4525-7513-1 (e)

Balboa Press rev. date: 06/05/2013

"I alone cannot change the world, but I can cast a stone across the waters to create many ripples."
—Mother Theresa

"The beauty of a lake reflects the beauty around it. When your mind is still, the beauty of the self is seen reflected in it."—BKS Iyengar

The Lake

The water,

a perfect mirror,

of colored trees and clouded sky.

Across the lake, in formation, birds fly.

Raindrops now trickle

sending separate

tiny ripples, tiny ripples.

m.a.g.

Like the rippling of the raindrops on water, I offer my reflections on the practice of yoga. While this offering is more suggestive than didactic I am inviting you to sample and reflect with me on some of the wisdom and ideology of this ancient practice.

When I was seventeen I was reading one of my favorite authors Herman Hesse. The book that ignited my imagination was Siddhartha. A phrase that stood out and seemed to resonate inside me:

> "Within you there is a stillness
> a sanctuary to which you can
> retreat at anytime and be yourself."
>
> Herman Hesse

A desire welled within me as I wondered if I too could know or understand this 'stillness' the author described. Simultaneously, my sister invited me to attend a yoga class with her. I recall the teacher saying to me I was natural at yoga. We exchanged smiles. She ended the class with the salutation 'Namaste.' To paraphrase the meaning, 'the light or spirit within me, salutes the light or spirit within you.' A seed was planted as I felt drawn to practice yoga.

I found myself repeatedly returning to practice yoga and with each return my gratitude deepened. My knowledge expanded as I quenched my thirst for a deeper understanding of yoga through books, audio, video tapes and the computer. After many years and many classes I decided I wanted to share this practice with others; with great humility I now teach yoga.

My style of teaching is remaining open and approachable to people who express an interest in yoga. I supply my classes with handouts compiled from a variety of books. While sifting through the vast knowledge and wisdom of yoga I sought to pare it down to be simply stated and easily applied. As a teacher the three ideologies that seem to stand out to me personally: Breathe, Move, Meditate.

"For those who have an intense urge for spirit and wisdom, it sits near them waiting."—Patanjali

BREATHE

"Breath is the bridge which connects life to consciousness which unites your body with your thoughts. Whenever your mind becomes scattered, use your breath to take hold of your mind again."
—Thich Nhat Hanh

Moving into my breath
I drift more deeply
savoring the stillness
the calm and peace
that is the truth.
Equanimity.

m.a.g.

1

Prana—The Breath: Yogis demonstrated great reverence for the breath as they observed that without the breath there is no life. The Sanskrit word prana is used for breathing exercises which translates as spirit-energy or life force. During my classes I instruct breathing exercises. I feel the following practices are most helpful for students.

Breathing Exercises

The following breathing practices will assist to slow your heart rate and lower your blood pressure.

Observing the Flow of Your Breath: Begin observing the flow of your breath using your imagination. As you breathe in, feel the coolness of your breath on the back of your throat: Imagine your breath like an elevator moving down below your navel as you breathe in: As you breathe out, you will feel the breath warm on the back of your throat and imagine the elevator moving up from your navel to the back of your throat as you exhale. Focus on the sensation of the coolness and the warmth of your breath. Practice 3 to 15 minutes.

<u>Breath Counting</u>: Inhale 1-2-3-4. Pause or hold your breath 1-2-3-4-5-6-7. Exhale 1-2-3-4-5-6-7-8. Repeat 8 times.

Observe the influence of your breath soothing your body and stilling your mind.

MOVE

Gramma's Wisdom
("Don't let the bed get you")

As a young adult I rented the upstairs apartment from my then-octogenarian grandmother. My grandmother kept her home spotlessly clean and baked homemade bread weekly. Marveling at her motivation and discipline, I asked, "Gramma, how do you do it? What's your secret?" She said, shaking her index finger at me, "Mary Ann, don't let the bed get you." I responded, "Huh? What does that mean?" She said, "When you wake up and think you have aches, pains, and worries and you want to stay in bed, don't let the bed get you. Instead, get up, start moving, make your work and before you know it, you will forget all about your aches, pains, and worries."

"Be like a branch of a tree; flex your body to face 'wind of sorrow;' flex little harder to dance in the wind of happiness."—Santosh Kalwar

"Joy is the expression of movement without interruption; the freedom of expression without judgment."—Unknown

"Everything in the universe has a rhythm; everything dances."—Maya Angelou

Wayne Dyer writes that "When you change the way you look at things, the things you look at change." Might I invite you to follow first by changing your perception of the way you look at exercise. For myself, like most people, the thought of exercise seems to imply some sort of sweat and/or drudgery. Marsha Doble writes, "I have to exercise this morning before my brain figures out what I'm doing." Mark Twain wrote, "I'm pushing sixty—that's enough exercise for me."

Instead, we will call it movement. Movement nurtures the body. When we move, there is an increase of endorphins to the brain and there is an increase of oxygen to the blood and organs. Mike Dooley stated, "When you move, the universe moves. When you stretch, it stretches. But always you must go first." Think like a dancer: Movement is participating in the dance of life. Isadora Duncan described dance as follows: "The dance is love, it is only love, and that is enough . . . I, then, it is amorously that I dance; to poem, to music, but now I would no longer like to dance to anything but the rhythm of my soul." As the dancer Martha Graham stated, "The body says what words cannot" and "Dance is the song of the body, either joy or pain" and further that "There is a vitality, a life force, a quickening, that is translated through you into action and because there is only one of you in all time this expression is unique."

One might experiment to find movement that feels pleasant and natural. When you do this, you will be gifting yourself with so many benefits (as I have with yoga). Oprah Winfrey stated, "Every day brings a chance for you to draw in breath, kick off your shoes, and dance." Author Alice Walker wrote, "Some say even to walk is a dance." Carol Welch defined movement, "Movement is a medicine for creating change in a person's physical, emotional, and mental states."

"Both man and air are purified by movement." —Proverb

"Asanas attune the body to meditation just as the guitar is tuned before a performance."—Unknown.

Asanas–Postures

The Eastern approach toward exercise or movement develops one's awareness through observation and tuning into one's own intuition. It is often exemplified by the lotus flower opening one petal at a time. Alternately, one is moving and resting, noticing the effects, the sensations in one's own body as the asanas are practiced. As Liz Lark wrote in her book *1,001 Pearls of Yoga Wisdom*, "Resting between asanas allows you to become more receptive in your yoga, as it gives time for both your body and your mind to process the effects, whether physical, mental, or emotional, of each movement."

When one synchronizes the breath together with movement one is creating a dialogue between the mind and the body. With continued practice of the asanas, one opens to achieve greater mind/body harmony.

"Yoga is 99% practice and 1% theory and our uniquely human capacity of connecting movement with breath and spiritual meaning. Yoga is born."
—K Pattabhi Jois

"Yoga is like music: the rhythm of the body, the melody of the mind, and the harmony of the soul create the symphony of life."—BKS Iyengar.

The Benefits of Practicing Yoga

The benefits include an increase in flexibility, range of motion, muscle tone, body awareness and deep breathing. There is a decrease in stress as it creates a feeling of calm, the breathing promotes the relaxation response in the body. Yoga also is beneficial in relieving back pain and osteoarthritis in the knees.

"It is through your body that you realize you are a spark of divinity."—BKS Iyengar.

Here's a sample of a relaxing sequence of asanas to try.

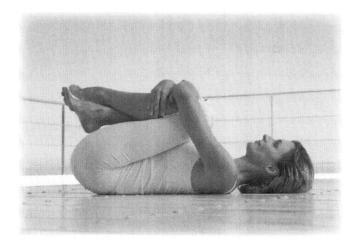

The curl: While lying on your back, bend your knees raising your feet. Wrap your arms around your legs, hugging your legs towards your chest. Exhale. Lift your head towards your knees. Inhale. Lower your head back to the floor. Repeat three times.

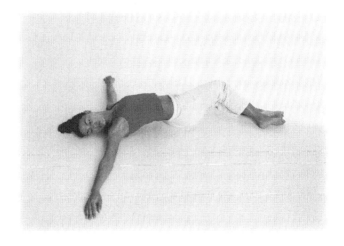

Spinal twist: Drop your arms parallel to your shoulder in a T-position. Keeping your knees bent, feet off the floor, roll at your hips to the left. Rest your legs on the floor. Turn your head to the right and hold four breaths. Roll at the hips to the right and turn your head to the left. Hold four breaths. Repeat three times each side.

Alternate arm and leg stretch: Lying on your back, raise your left leg hip height, point your toes to the wall below your foot. Inhaling, raise your left arm over your head, parallel with your shoulder. Reach with your fingers for the wall above your head. While stretching with your toes, reach for the opposite wall and take a deep breath and as you exhale, lower your arm back to your side and your leg back to the floor. Repeat three times on each side of your body.

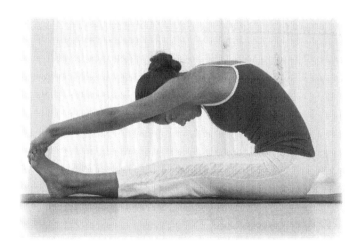

Sitting forward bend: Roll up into a sitting position to practice sitting forward bend. Inhale, bringing your arms over your head. As you exhale, lower your arms to your legs. Tuck your chin. Lower your head and hold this position for four breaths. Repeat three times.

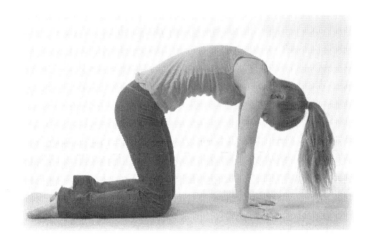

Cat/Cow: Continue as you kneel on all fours into tabletop position to begin practicing the cat asana. Kneeling on all fours, hands under your shoulders, knees under your hips, head parallel to the floor. Inhale as you lift your chin and tailbone up toward the ceiling.

Exhale and round your back toward the ceiling and tuck your chin towards your chest and tuck your tailbone. Repeat for eight breaths.

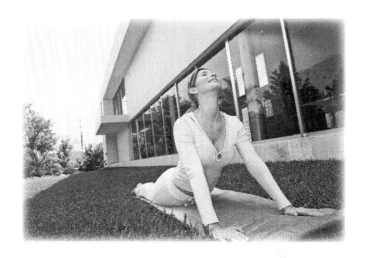

The Serpent: Next, slide your legs out from under your hips, lowering down onto your belly to practice the serpent asana. Place your elbows under your shoulders, forearms straight out. Position your legs about a hip distance apart and straighten at the elbows as you inhale. Hold for four breaths. Repeat three times.

Simply lower your head to your forearms, resting on your belly for eight breaths. Finally, roll onto your back and assume the corpse (or sponge) position.

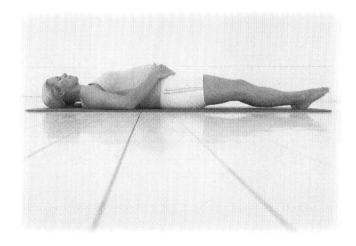

Shavasana: This pose is often referred to as sponge or corpse pose. It is during this asana that one lies still and allows the body to relax and the mind to become quiet.

"Relaxation is the prerequisite for that inner expression that allows a person to express the source of inspiration and joy within."—Deepak Chopra.

MEDITATE

"The flowering of love is meditation."—Jiddau Krishnamurti.

"If we sit with an increasing stillness of the body and attune our mind to the sky or to the ocean or to the myriad of stars at night or any other indicators of vastness, the mind gradually stills and the heart is filled with quiet joy."—Ravi Ravinda.

To gaze at the sunset, the clouds drifting while

listening to leaves rippling with the wind,

inside exists

a deep sense

of appreciation for the

palette of creation

and for a moment

time

stands

still.

m.a.g.

Meditation is a tool one can use to center calm and explore the inner self.

The following is a definition of meditation, according to medical-dictionary.thefreedictionary.com: "Meditation is a practice of concentrated focus upon a sound, object, visualization, the breath, movement, attention itself to increase awareness of the present moment, to reduce stress, promote relaxation, and enhance personal and spiritual growth."

There are a variety of meditation techniques available that one can practice. Often mantras accompany or can be added to the practice of meditation. For example, chanting "om" or "aum" during meditation aids in creating a deeper, more concentrated focus during the meditative process. Sri Chimnoy wrote, "Meditation gives us peace of mind without a tranquilizer, the peace of mind that we get from meditation does not fade away, it lasts for good in some corner of the inmost recesses of one's aspiring heart." Author Pema Chodon stated, "Meditation is not about trying to throw ourselves away and become something better, it's about befriending who we are."

"The soul never thinks without a picture."
—Aristotle.

"Creative visualization may be described as an extended meditation session that reaches beyond passive contemplation and achieves transformative action. The uses to which it may be applied are limited only by an individual's imagination."—Aberjhaini.

Guided imagery or guided meditation is a method used to assist one's imagination using verbal suggestions to create a relaxed yet focused state of mind. The most frequently used example of imagery is that of tasting a lemon. This demonstrates the connection between the mind and the body. Some benefits of guided imagery meditation include a decrease in blood pressure, stress, and pain; a sense of health; and an increase of optimism and self-esteem.

In Deepak Chopra's "Guided Meditation for Happiness" series, Deepak Chopra prefaced a guided meditation stating, "We will be guided in our attention on the more divine qualities of love, gratitude, compassion, ecstasy, peace, and equanimity. In this expanded state, the immune system is strengthened as the body repairs the damage caused by toxic experiences, relationships, environments, and substances."

I often facilitate this practice at the end of my classes while the class is resting in Sharvasana position. The following are examples of guided meditations you can practice.

While lying in Sharvasana, begin by using progressive relaxation. Bring your awareness to your feet. Flexing your feet, inhale, holding the tension and your breath for the count of eight and as you exhale, release the tension and release the breath. Moving your attention to your legs, inhale, tensing your legs, holding your breath for the count of eight, and exhaling, release the breath and the tension. Move your attention to your abdomen and your buttocks, tighten your muscles and inhale holding your breath for the count of eight and exhaling, feeling the sensation of tension melting down the lower limbs of the body, all the way down to the heels of your feet.

On the next inhale, tighten the chest, the back, and the belly, holding the breath for the count of eight. Exhaling, feeling the chest melt into the back, release the tension. Move your awareness to your upper limbs. Squeeze your hands into fists. Tighten the muscles from the fists up your arms to your shoulders. Inhale, raise your arms, holding your breath for the count of eight. As you exhale, dropping your arms back to the floor, allow the sensation of tension to melt from the shoulders down the arms to the wrists to the fingertips. Bring your attention to your head. Inhale, lift your head, squeeze the muscles in your face, clench your jaw, holding for the count of eight. As you exhale, lower your head back to the floor, releasing the tension in the neck, the head, the face, relaxing the forehead, the eyes, the cheeks, dropping your mouth open, letting go of the tension in the mouth and jaw. Bring your awareness to your breath as you allow yourself to become more and more at rest. Bring your awareness into your imagination . . .

Refer to progressive relaxation while assuming the Sponge position to enhance each guided meditation

Colored Clouds Meditation (Resting and healing with color): Imagine yourself lying on top of a grassy hill with the sun blanketing and warming your body. Breathing in, you feel warm and restful as you can hear the leaves rustling on the trees. As you look up at the blue sky, you notice the clouds are the colors of the rainbow. You see red, orange, yellow, green, blue, indigo, and violet clouds floating on the wind. To your surprise, one cloud is drifting towards you (pause). Notice the color of the cloud. You feel the cloud enveloping your whole body and lifting you. You know this cloud is a healing cloud. You feel all the muscles of your body sinking into the cloud, becoming more and more relaxed. The cloud is blanketing you from head to toe as you allow yourself to sink into the cloud as if it is a great feathered cushion. You can feel yourself drifting and floating, drifting and floating. The color of the cloud forms a mist. As you breathe in the mist, you feel the mist moving into your body, soothing, calming, healing you from the top of your head to the tips of your toes. Breathing and relaxing as you feel yourself drifting and floating, drifting and floating, feeling warmed and soothed as you allow yourself to become more and more at rest, breathing in, feeling peaceful and restored. The cloud returns you back to the hill and you watch it drift back into the sky. You release the images, returning back to the present, feeling refreshed and renewed.

The Garden of Your Heart Meditation: While in this relaxed state, focusing on your breath, move into your imagination. See yourself walking on a winding path. This is a path leading to the garden of your own heart. Looking down at your feet, noticing the path, ask yourself: Is it grassy? Is it a stone-path? Mosaics or tiles? You find yourself at a gate, and as you open the latch, you step into a beautiful garden. You are here to remove any weeds from the garden of your heart. Kneeling down, you begin to pull the weeds of sadness, sorrow, regret, anger, frustration, fear, and disappointment. You notice, as you remove the weeds, you feel a sense of peace moving into your heart-space. Breathe into your heart (pause). You feel the richness of the soil as you run your fingers through the earth. You begin to plant seeds of peace, love, laughter, and harmony. You see yourself patting atop the soil, covering the seeds. Breathing in, feeling a sense of peace and gratitude filling your heart, allowing yourself to bask in that sensation (pause), release the images, walking back on your path, returning to the present moment, maintaining a sense of peace and gratitude in your heart.

Memories of Love: Allowing yourself to relax, breathe and move into your memories. Opening yourself to those memories, allow yourself to recall those memories in your life when you felt safe, protected, and loved. It is as if you are opening a book of photographs. You may see memories of family gatherings, or friends. Allow yourself to be in that special place of love. Smell the aromas. Listen to the sounds. Soak in the sensation of love. Breathe it in, feeling a deep sense of gratitude for the blessings of love you have received in your life (pause). Close the book of photographs and return to the present moment with the knowledge of being loved, holding that sense of gratitude within your own heart.

The Wishing Tree: Breathe in and allow yourself to move into your imagination. Picture yourself walking along a path. You feel warmed by the sun and there is a cool breeze blowing through your hair. You take a deep breath and hear the birds singing. The sky is pale blue. The grass is an emerald green with bright specks of yellow dandelions swaying in the wind. You feel a calm sense of joy growing as you are on your way to the garden of wishes. You see a clearing through the trees. Walk up to a gate and as you open the latch, you see winding brick paths and beautiful flowers all around you. You are drinking in the colors with your eyes. The air is filled with the fragrant scent of the flowers. At the center of the garden, you see the magical wishing tree. You sit on the bench beside the tree, closing your eyes, breathing in all the beautiful scents filling the air. Next to you, there is a pen and paper. You begin to write your wishes on the paper one by one, feeling a sense of joyful anticipation as you write. You take your wishes and attach them to the tree. Feeling complete, you follow the path back to the gate. As you walk back, you are filled with hope and positive expectancy, imagining your wishes fulfilled (pause). Take a deep and clearing breath, open your eyes and bring yourself back into the present moment.

Your Retreat: Imagine yourself walking to your own personal retreat. As you walk, you gaze up, noticing the sun's rays shining in a splay of light through the leafy green trees. The air is warm and you hear the birds singing as they flit from branch to branch, tree to tree. Your retreat may be beside an ocean, a lake, on a mountain or hill, any place to which you feel intuitively drawn. The path widens and your step quickens to the porch of this special place. You open the door. As you look around the room, you see familiar objects and pictures of those you love placed around the room. You feel a deep sense of relief as you know this is the place where you go to rest and restore yourself. You take off your shoes and allow yourself to sink into the cushions of the couch. Take a deep breath, feel all tension melting from your body as you allow yourself to sink more deeply into the cushions. Beside you is a pen and paper. As you lie comfortably content, you see, on the left side of the paper, repeated words "I am fortunate because _____". You begin to write, filling in the page, "I am fortunate because _____". As you continue to write, you feel a deep sense of love and gratitude warming your heart and mind. A smile curls the corner of your mouth. You place the pen and paper aside, closing your eyes, reflecting more deeply, feeling more and more at peace, breathing in to this deep state of warmth and peace (pause). When you feel complete, take a deep clearing breath, coming back into the present, feeling refreshed and renewed.

Meeting Your Guardian Angel: Imagine you are walking down a path. It is a beautiful spring day. The trees are blossoming with white, pink and purple flowers. The sun is shining, the birds are singing, and a path leads you to a garden. In the center of the garden, you see a pond. The sun sparkles like diamonds on the surface of the water as waves ripple the water of the pond. You see a white gazebo and sit quietly reflecting on the beauty of the pond. Your angel quietly sits beside you. You reach your hand over and feel the angel's reassuring touch. You begin to open your heart to your angel, expressing any concerns you have, feeling a deep sense of trust, knowing your angel will assist you and guide you. Taking a deep breath, feeling a sense of peace and comfort; your angel knows the quality you need to assist you on your path. He/she places a box in your hand and leaves the garden. You open the box and you see the quality. It may be patience, love, understanding, flexibility, simplicity, gratitude, truth, humor, grace. You know this is magical and you open your heart to receive the quality that you have been gifted. Invoke and breathe the gift, the quality, into your heart (pause). When you feel complete, you leave the garden, returning to the present, feeling fulfilled.

"Wake at dawn with a winged heart and give thanks for another day."—Kahlil Gibran.

ADD GRATITUDE DAILY

"Gratitude is not only the greatest of all virtues, but the parent of all others."—Marcus Tillius Cicero.

"What I learned is there's a scientifically proven phenomenon that's attached to gratitude and that if you consciously take note of what's good in your life, qualifiable benefits happen."—Deborah Norville.

Research has been conducted at the University of California to measure the value of practicing gratitude in your life. Robert Emmons is considered to be a world leader in studying the effects of gratitude. The study included people from the ages of 8 to eighty. People were asked to maintain gratitude journals for three weeks; the participants recorded consistently a variety of positive benefits. Studies have demonstrated this practice improves your health physically, psychologically, and socially. Some inclusive benefits noted are: stronger immune systems, decrease in blood pressure, increase in positive emotions and optimism, increase in compassion, and a decrease in feeling lonely and/or isolated. More information is available as Robert Emmons has authored a book *Thanks. How the New Science of Gratitude Can Make You Happier.*

"Gratitude is the creative force; the mother and father of love. It is in gratitude that real love exists. Love expands when gratitude is there."—Sri Chinmoy.

Gratitude is exemplified in this poem by Ralph Waldo Emerson:

'For each morning with its light

For rest and shelter of the night

For health and food, for love and friends

For everything thy goodness sends.'

It is with gratitude that I have shared my thoughts and insights on the practice of yoga. As Elizabeth Kubler Ross stated, "There's no need to go to India or anywhere to find peace. You will find that deep place of silence within your room, your garden, or even your bathtub."

My hope is to encourage and inspire you to breathe deeply, move joyously, and meditate gratefully.

> "Hope is the thing with feathers,
> that perches in the soul
> and sings the tune without words
> and never stops at all."
>
> Emily Dickinson

Remember my Gramma's advice: Don't let the bed get you.

Thank you to the universe for the blessing of words pouring from pen to paper while writing this book. Thank you to the yogis past and present for their truth and wisdom. Thank you to my students who have been a great source of love and support. I would like to thank my daughter Jocelyn and my granddaughter Cassadi for their love, patience and support, as well as my family and friends. And a special thank you to Matthew Niemiec for his continual confidence and encouragement.